Autophagy

Keto and Fasting Secrets You Need for Extreme Weight Loss and Anti-Aging - Heal Your Body from Within

<u>Disclaimer Notice:</u>

Please note the information contained within this document is for educational and entertainment purposes only. All effort has been executed to present accurate, up to date, and reliable, complete information. No warranties of any kind are declared or implied. Readers acknowledge that the author is not engaging in the rendering of legal, financial, medical or professional advice. The content within this book has been derived from various sources. Please consult a licensed professional before attempting any techniques outlined in this book.

By reading this document, the reader agrees that under no circumstances is the author responsible for any losses, direct or indirect, which are incurred as a result of the use of information contained within this document, including, but not limited to, — errors, omissions, or inaccuracies.

Table of Contents

Introduction

People are always on the lookout for trends that can help them stay fit and healthy. There are various marketing gimmicks and weight loss processes that hit markets regularly. Some of these work very well while others are a complete fad.

If you want to stay healthy, it is important to incorporate the right weight loss or health management techniques that help you to look great and feel great from within.

Autophagy is a scientific method that works well to protect your body and the cells from cellular damage. This helps with reversing the signs of aging and making you feel and look a lot younger. This is a cytoplasmic catabolic process that controls cellular damage and also enhances faster tissue and cell repair.

Apart from the visible benefits you can receive by adapting to an autophagy way of life, you also reverse the signs of aging internally. This means you are less prone to suffer from age-related diseases. Not only will you look good externally, but you your internal organs will also be functioning to the maximum potential. This creates a feel-good factor, and it helps in various aspects of life as well.

So how exactly do you get yourself hooked on to the autophagy way of life? It's simple. There are few dietary restrictions you have to keep in mind, and you have to make minor changes in your lifestyle so you can lead a healthy and fruitful life.

If you're looking to lose weight and stay in shape but you are also concerned about your health and you want to provide your body with the right nourishment, autophagy is something you should incorporate into your life. From learning how to control what you eat to getting in shape and feeling healthy about yourself, autophagy has it all! This guide will help you discover the amazing secrets of autophagy and how you can benefit from it.

Chapter 1: Autophagy, What Is It?

You may have heard the term autophagy a lot, and this book will give you a better understanding of its concept and how it benefits your body. Autophagy is derived from two Greek words *auto* and *phagy*. *Auto* means "self" and *phagy* means "eating." This method requires some eating habits that you need to develop in order for your body to stay healthy. In the process of autophagy, the habit of eating right is important in order to repair the damaged cells in your body.

When new cells are formed, the old cells are destroyed. Autophagy helps in the process of degradation of old cells and the formation of new ones. In simple words, autophagy is nothing but a process that helps to clean out the damaged cells in the body for better functionality. This cleansing enhances the healing process and helps the body healthy.

Apoptosis

While autophagy includes the regeneration of cells within the body, there are also a number of cells that are killed. The process of programmed cell death is called apoptosis. Apoptosis basically keeps track of all the healthy cells in the body and destroys the cells that are damaged or unnecessary. With the help of autophagy, some cells are able to survive stress. This stress can be in two forms—one would be external stress caused by the lack of nutrients the body receives, and the other would be internal stress, which is caused by the accumulation of the damaged cells or any kind of invasion by an infective organism.

The Secret of Autophagy

Not a lot of people know this, but autophagy can help cleanse your body in no time. Gone are the days when you had to depend on detox diets as well as juice cleanses to get rid of the toxins from your body. These processes do not help the body in any way and will only prolong your recovery process.

We're not saying it's wrong to drink kale juices or flush out toxins from your body. All we're saying is autophagy will help you flush out these toxins faster than anything else even if you don't include a bitter juice to your routine.

There is one small fact most people are not aware of, and that is self-cannibalism. Self-cannibalism is nothing but training the body to eat itself. As bad as it may sound, this is not some kind of flesh-eating disease that will take away your life.

It is the process of autophagy, which will kill the dead cells in the body and regenerate new ones to help increase the metabolism rate and destroy the toxins in the body. As stated above, autophagy in Greek means self-eating. This is the body's natural way of cleaning the system. There are a number of dead cells and scrap formed in the body over a period of time, and autophagy helps remove these cell membranes and dead cells and replaces them with new cells.

"Autophagy makes us more efficient machines to get rid of faulty parts, stop cancerous growths, and stop metabolic dysfunction like obesity and diabetes."[1]

---

[1] Colin Champ, MD, board-certified radiation oncologist, assistant professor at the University of Pittsburgh Medical Center and author of the renowned book *Misguided Medicine*.

This recycling process that the body undergoes helps clean it very effectively. It also helps control the immunity as well as the inflammation in the body. Scientists have conducted studies on lab rats that were not capable of autophagy, and they found that these rats were always sleepy, had high cholesterol, had put on a lot of weight, and had impaired brains. Over a period of time, if your body does not clear out the toxins, this is exactly what will happen to the internal system, and your body will end up suffering. As someone rightly said, autophagy is nature's anti-aging process, and you can help improve this process with three effective methods.

Exercise Regularly

Have you ever noticed that your body pains a lot and you end up sweating a lot after you have worked out? Have you ever wondered why this happens? When you work out or exercise regularly, it damages your muscles. This damage causes microscopic tears, and the body rushes to heal this damage. When the body does this over and over again, the muscles start growing stronger, and it will not suffer any more damage. This is the reason people keep saying you need to exercise regularly. If you exercise once a month, your muscles will keep getting damaged. While your body will repair the damage every time this happens, your muscles will never become immune to the damage if you do not exercise regularly.

Exercising every day or at least thrice a week will ensure your body cleanses itself from within. Every person is different, and you need to figure out the extent to which you need to exercise and how much needs to be done every day in order for your body to heal properly. If you go beyond your capacity, your muscles will break down, and your body may not be able to heal those muscles in time. This is what causes muscle tear as well as muscle pulls on some occasions.

Fasting

Fasting is another efficient way of cleansing your system from within. It may sound weird, but when you eat, it goes against the principle of autophagy. Until your body is stressed and there are some internal or external factors affecting it, the process of autophagy will not be as efficient as you'd like it to be. When you put your body through the stress of skipping meals, your body may not enjoy the process, but it will begin to benefit from it eventually.

Fasting occasionally has a number of benefits, and in some cases, it has shown to reduce the risk of heart disease as well as diabetes. This is because the process of autophagy becomes efficient in the body. In certain cases, autophagy has helped lower the risk of various brain-related diseases, such as Parkinson's and Alzheimer's.

Lowering the Intake of Carbs

Eating irregular meals and fasting once a month are things almost everyone can do. While there are people who can fast regularly, there are others who simply can't give up tasty food made by their family every day. There is another way your body can benefit without having to give up on any of your favorite foods. This process is called ketosis.

Ketosis is very popular, especially among bodybuilders and among people that are looking to live a long healthy life. The key to ketosis is to reduce the carbs you consume.

When you start doing this, your body will have no option but to use the fats in your body as a source of fuel.

Ketosis is a brilliant way of retaining muscle in the body and losing body fat in no time. Some people have even called ketosis as an autophagy hack. This is because you get the same benefits of autophagy without the need to fast. A recent study has also shown that epileptic children that followed the ketosis diet reduced their seizures by almost 50 percent. The ketosis diet is very high in fat as well as protein, and the carbs are kept to the bare minimum.

Chapter 2: The Benefits of Autophagy

Autophagy, which is also referred to as self-eating, is a method that enables you to restore damaged cells and help to heal your body from within. This is a scientifically proven method that not only works well in weight management but also has various other benefits that help your body to stay healthy and young. If you are looking for a solution to keep yourself fit and rejuvenated, then it is always advisable to use natural methods that do not involve any antibiotic and have proven results to back them up. The best part about relying on autophagy is that it works effectively to make your body stronger and increases your immunity. This enables you to fight infections and clean up cells more regularly. If you have heard a lot about autophagy but you are not too sure what it has in store for you, then here are a few things about autophagy you need to know about.

1. Autophagy May Save Your Life

While this statement may sound extreme, it is actually true and scientifically proven. Autophagy helps you to lead a healthy and more fruitful life. This enhances your overall lifestyle and makes you stronger. The process of autophagy, which has been known for many years, helps preserve life in the worst of situations. If you have been suffering from a lot of stress and you have succumbed to a number of infections, it's the best time for you to adapt to autophagy. It works really well in repairing the cells in your body with minimum damage. If you want autophagy to work perfectly well for your body, then you may want to try combining it with intermittent fasting. This is a form of fasting that provides the body with a little bit of fat to go through the day.

When you begin the process of autophagy, you take out intruders from your body, which include glucose and inflammation. Autophagy can reduce inflammation to a great extent. This helps reduce the number of times you fall sick as your immune system gets stronger. The process not only conserves your energy but also helps repair your cells effectively. Autophagy can also reduce the risk of cancer by protecting your cells and repairing them on time.

2. Autophagy May Improve the Quality and Length of Your Life

People spend a lot of money visiting salons and spas to reverse the signs of aging. Cosmetic surgeries like Botox have become more prominent because people want to look younger. What they don't realize is that when they start leading a healthier lifestyle and adapt to a natural process instead, the skin retains its elasticity naturally without any need for cosmetic surgery. Apart from skin-deep beauty, autophagy also enhances cellular health, making your body younger from within.

People constantly measure their chronological age and biological age to give them a clear picture of how healthy they actually are. Adapting to autophagy will help you reduce your chronological age and keep you healthy from within. When your body repairs cells faster, not only do you feel younger, but you also start looking a lot younger. Your energy levels will be higher than you've ever imagined, and you will start feeling much better. It's not uncommon to see people who are as young as thirty years get extremely tired when they walk up a flight of stairs. This isn't only because they are overweight but also because they are unhealthy from within, and it needs to be treated.

Losing weight isn't always the solution. While fat is bad for your body, getting healthy is what you need to start focusing on because that's what really matters. With autophagy not only do you manage to lose weight, but you also manage to get healthy.

3. Autophagy Helps Your Metabolism Work Better

Having a low metabolism rate is not great for your system because it means you are storing more fat in your body. With a low metabolism rate, even when you eat small meals, you start getting fat. Autophagy helps get out all the trash from your system, and this works well in various ways. Not only does it help to replace all the damaged cells in your body, but this process also works well to boost your metabolism rate. This is vital in order to have a healthy functioning system.

When your metabolism rates are higher, your body tends to burn fat faster. This means that you will make use of all the nutrients in your body in a better way. Higher metabolism rate lowers the risk of weight gain and also enhances digestion. This encourages the cells to work more effectively, keeping your body healthy and young. People who have office jobs and tend to sit for long hours usually suffer from low metabolism rates, and even when they try to control what they eat, they do not lose weight because the body tends to store whatever little fat they consume. This is what leads to an unhealthy lifestyle, and people start falling sick even at a young age.

4. Autophagy Reduces the Risk of Neurodegenerative Diseases

Neurodegenerative diseases are caused when protein starts accumulating around your brain cells because they are not functional. When this protein accumulation starts to increase, neurodegenerative problems begin to show up. Adapting to autophagy helps clean up your internal system, and this prevents the protein accumulation around your brain. This reduces the risk of this disease.

People who adapt to autophagy are less likely to suffer from Parkinson's disease and Alzheimer's disease. They are also less likely to suffer from memory-related problems. While some people believe that they do not need to adapt to autophagy because they are young and they won't suffer from neurodegenerative problems until they get older, the truth is that the onset of Alzheimer's and Parkinson's begins at a young age, and you won't even realize when it begins to affect you. The sooner you move to a healthier lifestyle, the healthier you stay, and the better it is for your brain health as well.

Apart from Alzheimer's and Parkinson's, dementia is also a popular neurodegenerative condition that occurs because of protein accumulation around the brain. Dementia is more popular with diabetic patients. Autophagy keeps diabetes in control, thereby lowering the risk of dementia considerably.

5. Autophagy Regulates Inflammation

Autophagy can reduce inflammation considerably because of the cell repair that it performs in your body. The inflammation in your body is reduced by a great deal, and your body is able to fight infectious diseases and stays strong. Autophagy also boosts your immune system, and you are less likely to fall sick. If you constantly suffer from a cold or cough, autophagy is a great way to limit the number of times you call in sick at work. It also makes you lead a fuller life without constantly worrying about your health. If you love travelling but allergens in the air make you fall sick, with autophagy you will now manage to go out more often with a reduced risk of falling sick.

6. Autophagy Fights Infectious Diseases

Apart from boosting the immune system, autophagy also works well to remove certain microbes from the body. Microbes are inside the cells and are the main cause of life-threatening diseases, including tuberculosis and HIV. While it doesn't eliminate these diseases from the system, it lowers the risk of one contracting them, and it fights them more effectively. It also manages to get rid of the dirty toxins that have started accumulating in your body. Autophagy can help treat your system and can keep it safe from an infection, especially the ones that go into your system through the food.

7. Autophagy Improves Muscle Performance

People who enjoy working out usually depend on artificial protein shakes and supplements to increase the size of their muscles. These supplements have a lot of side effects, and they can damage your body when used in the long term. If you want to increase the size of your muscles naturally, then adapting to autophagy is a healthier alternative. The best part about autophagy is that it has no side effects, and it helps your muscles to expand a lot faster. It's great for inflammation because it manages to soothe your muscles after an exercise. It also repairs muscle tissue effectively and increases your stamina so you perform more rigorously in the gym without having to suffer too much pain.

Autophagy also repairs dead tissues and damaged cells to make you feel healthy and more active. If you often feel tired and drained out once you get to the gym, once you begin autophagy, you will not feel this anymore because it increases your energy as well as your stamina.

8. Autophagy Prevents the Onset of Cancer

Chronic cell damage and inflammation are the leading reasons people suffer from cancer. The lifestyle people lead today also increases the chances of cancer. Adapting to autophagy not only reduces the chances of cancer but also protects the body against it. A strong immune system can work really well to keep cancer cells away.

Autophagy works well with regard to cell damage repair, and it also treats free radicals, which are the leading cause of cancer. People suffering from cancer can also benefit from adapting to autophagy in a great way. It works really well during chemotherapy sessions, and it enhances the treatment greatly by working with the medication to kill cancer cells. While there is no definite way to prove that autophagy can contribute toward the prevention of cancer completely, it definitely assists in reducing the risk as well as enhancing the treatment.

9. Autophagy Improves Your Digestive Health

Digestive health is vital in order for people to feel good from the inside and manage to keep a clear and healthy gut. Autophagy manages to repair the cells that line the gastrointestinal tract, thereby enhancing the performance of your digestive system. When the digestive cells are repaired more effectively, it helps the system to get rid of all the toxins that are ruining the system from within. This also contributes to better bowel movements and reduces inflammation in the bowel, which usually results in inconsistent schedules and a sick feeling because of constipation.

People who have very little activity in their lives tend to suffer from constipation because they have a lot of damaged cells in the gastrointestinal tract, and this prevents the digestive system from acting effectively. Once you adapt to autophagy, the cells will be repaired. This, in turn, works extremely well on your complete digestive system.

10. Autophagy Improves Your Skin Health

Dead skin cells make your skin look dull and tired, and they increase the signs of aging at an early age. If you want to have healthy skin, it is important for you to get rid of all these dead cells, and make sure that your skin does not lose its elasticity. Autophagy is an amazing technique to promote better skin health because it gets rid of all the damaged cells and takes out all the toxins from your skin, thereby making it glow and look radiant and clean. People who suffer from skin-related problems, like acne or infections on the skin, will also benefit from autophagy because it helps kill the bacteria that settle down on your skin. Autophagy will leave you with clean skin from within as well. Once you adapt to autophagy, you can forget about all those expensive skin creams and treatments that you've been investing in just so that you could cover up your skin problems. You'll have healthy skin that is low maintenance, and even when you wake up in the morning, you will still look as beautiful as ever.

11. Autophagy Can Help Maintain a Healthy Weight

One of the major reasons autophagy gains so much recognition around the globe is the fact that it can help maintain a healthy weight.

Since it helps boost your metabolism levels and reduces the unnecessary inflammation, it manages to keep your body healthy and enhances the fat-burning process. This results in a leaner body even if you don't have to spend a lot of time exercising. While it is recommended that you indulge in a little exercise every day to enhance autophagy, the process works even when you are sitting at your work desk because the process itself burns fat much faster than you've ever imagined.

12. Autophagy (Cell-Eating) Minimizes Apoptosis (Cell Death)

Apoptosis is called cell death, which is a little different in comparison to autophagy. While autophagy works toward treating and repairing the cells in your body, apoptosis kills them. It takes a lot of time for your body to create new cells, and repairing these cells is always a better way to deal with them. Your body also needs to generate a lot of energy in order to renew the cells, and that's why autophagy is a better solution because it minimizes apoptosis and prevents cell death completely.

Chapter 3: What Activates Autophagy?

There are a number of ways that you can increase the autophagy process in your body. The process can be activated in order to provide maximum benefit to your mind as well as your body. There are two ways that you can increase autophagy—one is by inducing a little bit of stress that will help activate autophagy, and the other is by ingesting something that will help activate it.

Stressing the Body

Stressing the body can be done in a couple of days. It can be in the form of exercise, or it can be in the form of fasting. While you can use either of these methods to activate autophagy, you should know that stressing the body requires a lot of discipline, and it needs to be done regularly in order for autophagy to be successful.

Activating through Ingestion

There are a number of things that you can do to activate autophagy artificially. It can be done by going on a particular diet or eating certain foods. There are also various remedies and supplements that are available that can help activate autophagy.

Apart from the above methods, there are also a number of lifestyle choices that you can make in order to increase autophagy. Let us look at the best methods to increase autophagy in your body.

Aerobic Exercise

A number of studies have shown that aerobic exercise can help activate autophagy in the brain as well as muscle tissues. This happens because of a lot of stress that is placed on the cells, and the stress automatically activates autophagy. There are a couple of benefits of aerobic exercise. One is it makes you feel fit and you will end up feeling great every day, and the other is you will be able to activate autophagy and make sure that the cells recover in your body on time.

Calorie Restriction and Intermittent Fasting

These are also two great methods to activate autophagy in your body. When you deprive your body of nutrients, it will help with the recycling of the cellular components. This will ensure that your cells function properly without any dependency from outside. Depriving your body of nutrients can be done in a couple of ways. You can choose to fast, or you can restrict your calorie intake. It is said that short-term fasting is the best way to activate autophagy and is the perfect way to fight neurological conditions.

Ketogenic Diet

As you are already aware, the ketogenic diet is nothing but the reduction of carbon intake and the increase of fat intake in the body. This forces the body to shift the energy use to ketones rather than glucose.

Sleep Well

Another factor that helps activate autophagy is sleep. Not a lot of people know this, but your biological clock actually has a huge impact on the autophagy rhythm of your body. When you do not get sufficient sleep, the autophagy process gets interrupted, and it will get negatively affected. There have been studies where sleep disruption has also caused the interruption of protein transmission in the body.

Drink Lots of Coffee

Among the foods that help activate autophagy, coffee is one of the best. Studies have proven that coffee helps increase autophagy and makes it extremely efficient. While there are studies that show that too much coffee does have adverse effects on one's health, you should know that the autophagy process does not really get affected by the intake of coffee.

Drink a Lot of Green Tea

As you are already aware, green tea has a number of benefits, and it helps protect the heart as well as keeps cancer away with the help of its antioxidants. Apart from these benefits, you should also know that green tea helps activate autophagy. There are a number of active ingredients in green tea that are supposedly the best when it comes to activating autophagy.

Coconut Oil Simulation

Another way to increase autophagy or to activate it is by consuming coconut oil. Like the other food items that help activate autophagy, coconut oil also has a number of benefits, and you should make it a part of your regular diet in order to get the maximum benefit out of it. Coconut oil helps increase autophagy by increasing the ketone levels in the body.

Ginger

Ginger has an active constituent that can also help to induce autophagy. Ginger blocks mTOR and increases the autophagy process in your body.

Galangal

Galangal is usually found in various dishes in Southeast Asia, and it is said to be an amazing ingredient that can help induce autophagy. It is said that galangin, the prime constituent of galangal, helps increase autophagy in the body.

Reishi Mushroom Extract

A number of people use reishi mushroom as part of their diet because of the health benefits that it provides. It is said that reishi mushrooms improve the immunity of the body and increase the autophagy process. Reishi mushroom extract also prevents colon cancer and breast cancer.

Resveratrol

When it comes to activation of autophagy with the help of supplements, resveratrol is not very far behind. Resveratrol is a very strong polyphenol and is usually found in wine, soy, grapes, and peanuts. When you consume resveratrol, you will be able to activate autophagy, and it provides a number of long-term benefits to the body.

Vitamin D

People use vitamin D supplements as part of their diet, and it is also beneficial to the skin when you are exposed to sunlight. Research has also proven that vitamin D increases autophagy and protects pancreatic cells. This is very therapeutic as far as diabetes is concerned.

Omega-3 and Omega-6 Fats

When it comes to omega-3 and omega-6 fats, there are a number of benefits that your body receives. These polyunsaturated fats can increase the lifespan of a person, and it can also activate the autophagy process in the body.

Ginseng

Ginseng is another supplement that helps activate autophagy in the body. This activation is caused by ginsenosides that you will find in ginseng.

Melatonin

For people that do not know, melatonin helps regulate your sleep cycles, and it also regulates the circadian rhythm. Melatonin also induces autophagy and protects you from various neuropsychiatric disorders as well as cancer.

Amla (Indian Gooseberry)

For people that live in Asia, you must be aware that amla has a number of health benefits, and it prevents a number of diseases. For those that have not seen or tasted an amla, you should know that it is also known as Indian gooseberry and it also helps activate autophagy in the body.

Chapter 4: Intermittent Fasting

Intermittent fasting is one of the best ways to activate autophagy. It is beneficial on its own as well as when combined with autophagy. In case you are wondering why you should start intermittent fasting, then it's important for you to know the amazing benefits that it has to offer.

Enhances Cell, Genes, and Hormone Functionality

Intermittent fasting is when you fast for a few hours before you eat something. There are several ways your body reacts to this situation, and here are a few things that help in cell and hormone functionality. When you starve for long intervals, your body focuses on cell repair, and it also boosts the hormones in the system, making fat storage more accessible.

When you fast for long hours, the insulin level in your body starts dropping significantly, and this enhances the fat-burning process, which is effective for weight loss and weight management. Fasting also enhances the human growth hormone, which helps in muscle gain. If you are focusing on increasing your muscle mass in the body, then fasting for long hours is definitely something that will help you. The minute you stop eating, your body's first reaction is to focus on cell repair, and this helps the system become healthy from within. It protects the genes in your system, and it also increases protection against a number of age-related diseases. People who suffer from hormonal imbalance can benefit greatly when they start intermittent fasting to activate autophagy. This is also a great solution for people with high diabetes because it helps regularize blood sugar levels.

Lose Weight

One of the major reasons why autophagy has gained so much popularity is because it is an effective weight loss process. If you're looking to lose weight but you don't have enough time to head to the gym and exercise or even follow a diet plan, then autophagy and intermittent fasting will benefit you in many ways. By compensating on the number of meals you eat, you give your body lesser calories, and this aids in weight loss.

Apart from the fewer calories you consume, intermittent fasting also works well to enhance the metabolism rate and hormonal functionality. This further improves the process of weight loss and helps you get slimmer and leaner a lot faster. Since it helps boost metabolism in your body, even with fewer meals, you will start to feel fuller, and your body will start cleansing itself more effectively. The smaller the size of your meals, the easier it is for your body to heal from within. It's not just the number of calories you consume but also the healing process, which includes cell repair, and increasing muscle mass through better hormonal function. If you have a low metabolism level, intermittent fasting is a great way to boost it.

Great for Diabetics

The risk of diabetes has increased greatly in recent years, and people as young as the age of twenty are suffering from high blood sugar levels because of the kind of lifestyle they lead. When sugar levels in the body keep on increasing, there are some people that develop insulin resistance or type 2 diabetes. This requires regular insulin injection to balance out the sugar level. Intermittent fasting enhances the blood sugar levels in the body and reduces the risk of insulin resistance, which helps your body produce insulin more effectively. It manages to regularize the blood sugar levels a lot better and keep diabetes in control.

People who suffer from diabetes are also prone to kidney diseases and skin infections. However, intermittent fasting can help to reduce these problems and keep your body healthier. People who suffer from high diabetes also tend to have low energy levels, but intermittent fasting can help boost their energy levels and make them feel more energetic during the course of the day. If you are struggling with getting work done regularly because of the way you feel, intermittent fasting is one of the best ways to start being more efficient and getting more done every day.

Reduce Stress and Inflammation

Not a lot of people know this, but oxidative stress can lead to a number of chronic diseases as well as increased premature aging in the body. Intermittent fasting lowers your stress levels and makes you feel more positive and motivated. It enhances cell repair and eradicates the free radicals in the body, which are linked to a number of diseases.

Regular intermittent fasting also fights inflammation, which is another cause of various diseases, including the common cold. Stress and inflammation are so common today. It makes a lot of sense to adapt to autophagy and intermittent fasting in order to seek health benefits in the long run.

Good for Your Heart

Intermittent fasting has been linked to heart protection as it lowers the risk of heart diseases. Heart diseases are ranked as the number-one killer all over the world, and not looking after your heart could be an invitation to a number of illnesses. This includes high cholesterol level and the risk of a heart attack. Intermittent fasting lowers cholesterol levels and inflammatory markers, along with the blood sugar level. This keeps your body healthy and lowers the risk of heart diseases considerably.

Can Help Lower the Risk of Cancer

Intermittent fasting has been linked with lowering the risk of cancer as well. Cancer is caused because of an uncontrolled growth of radical cells. Intermittent fasting helps repair cells, control free radicals, and eradicate the main cause of cancer. Regularly resorting to intermittent fasting can help to lower the risk of cancer by healing these cells a lot faster. People who suffer from cancer will also manage to get a lot of relief through intermittent fasting because it helps reverse the side effects of chemotherapy and enhances the results.

It's Great for Your Brain

A lot of people look at intermittent fasting as a way to heal the body. The truth is intermittent fasting works wonders not just for your body but also for your brain. It helps you increase the level of a protein called neurotrophic, which is the main reason for curbing depression and anxiety. Studies have shown that people who are relatively less stressed are also less likely to suffer from brain-related diseases. Intermittent fasting can also help to protect against brain damage and lower the risk of strokes.

Chapter 5: Keto Diet

The keto diet has gained a lot of popularity over the past years. A keto diet plan includes eating food that is high in fat but low in carbs. This converts your body into a fat-burning machine that enhances weight loss a lot faster. When your keto diet is combined with autophagy, it works wonders to help you slim down and look great. There are various reasons that a number of celebrities have turned toward the keto diet and have begun incorporating its principles.

What Is a Keto Diet?

The fundamental principle of the keto diet is that it converts the food you consume into energy, and this enhances the fat-burning process to help you tone down. By consuming very little carbohydrates, your body suffers from a metabolic shock, and it starts burning fat for fuel instead of carbohydrates. Since your body doesn't get any carbohydrates, it starts turning fatty acids into ketones, which is known as an alternative source of energy in the body. Apart from helping in weight loss, it is also a great way to reduce inflammation in the body and lower the blood sugar level, which makes it a great alternative for people with high sugar in the body.

While the keto diet has gained a lot of popularity recently, this diet has actually been around for almost a century. It was primarily used to treat people that suffered from epilepsy in the 1920s. This diet is still highly effective for epileptic patients who do not respond to well to medications.

Health Benefits of the Keto Diet

Burns Fat

The primary benefit of a keto diet is that it helps you to lose weight effectively and quickly. Since your body stops consuming carbohydrates, it uses the fatty acids to form an alternate form of energy to fuel the body, and this causes it to start burning a lot of fat. The keto diet plan is also very effective to help curb your appetite because it can help you to go without food for long hours. If you have a lot of stubborn fat in your body, the keto diet is perfect for you because this diet forces your body to get into the deepest part and use the fat for energy.

Boost Your Immune System

While the keto diet burns a lot of fat in your body, it doesn't make you weak in any way. The diet plan is designed in a way to assist your body get stronger and reduce information to a great extent. A recent research has proven that people that follow a keto diet tend to fall sick less often as compared to those who follow other diet plans.

Nourishes Your Brain

One of the best things about a keto diet is that it provides your brain with a lot of energy by limiting the carb intake. Fat is one of the best ways to keep your brain strong. Since 60 percent of the brain is fat, in order for your brain to continue functioning smoothly, it's good to provide the brain with enough fat regularly. Your brain comprises of various fats, which include omega-3, which is used to develop the brain, and saturated fat, which works as an insulation layer around the brain, keeping the neurons strong and ensuring that you do not suffer from any brain-related problems.

Increases Energy

One of the major problems with most diet plans is that it becomes difficult for people to perform effectively during the day. People who lead a hectic life seldom manage to follow a diet plan because they need a certain amount of energy and the diet plan makes them feel lethargic and tired. The best thing about following a keto diet plan is that it provides you with a lot of energy, thereby keeping you active throughout the day. This is a great form of autophagy because ketosis is known to power you and give you spurts of energy at regular intervals.

What Can You Eat When on a Keto Diet?

A keto diet usually consists of high-fat food. You can include small amounts of proteins and carbohydrates as well, depending on what meal plan you choose. Ideally, 75 percent of your meal plan should consist of fat, and 20 percent should consist of protein. The remaining 5 percent of your diet can comprise of carbs, but then again, you can also choose to eliminate carbohydrates completely from your diet.

There are four kinds of keto diet plans:

- Standard

- Cyclical

- Targeted

- Dirty

Standard Keto Diet Plan

The standard diet plan is popular among most

keto dieters because it's easy to follow and convenient. With this diet plan, you need to consume very little carbohydrates during the day or eliminate them completely if possible. Someone on a keto diet should consume nothing more than fifty grams of carbohydrates per day. While this may seem like an impossible task, there are a number of dieters who manage to consume as little as twenty grams of carbohydrate in a day and still pull through the day with a lot of energy.

Cyclical Keto Diet Plan

This is what people call a cheat keto diet plan. In this diet plan, you need to follow the standard keto diet plan for five days of the week, and on the sixth and seventh day, you can consume up to 150 grams of carbohydrates. It's called a cycle of consuming carbohydrates every week in order to reduce the negative effects that a lot of people may face while suddenly eliminating carbohydrates from their diet. While it is not common for keto diet followers to fall ill, in rare cases, people may enhance their thyroid or suffer from dry eyes if they eliminate carbohydrates completely. If you have thyroid problems, it is always advisable to follow the cyclical keto diet plan.

Targeted Keto Diet Plan

This diet is similar to the standard keto diet plan, except you can eat carbohydrates about thirty minutes before you work out. This diet plan only works for people who spend at least five days a week in the gym and put a lot of energy into exercising. The glucose that carbohydrates release helps boost performance during an exercise session, which is why gym goers can consider using this diet plan.

Dirty Keto Diet Plan

A dirty keto diet plan includes the same amount of fat, protein, and carbohydrates like a standard keto diet, except for the fact that you don't need to keep a count of the calories you consume. This means you can have a large chicken salad and a diet Pepsi just before you hit the hay.

The important thing for people to understand is that every diet plan is different. Not all of them will work as effectively for you as they do for another person. You need to figure out which keto diet plan suits your body the best.

List of Foods to Avoid While on a Keto Diet

The best thing about a keto diet is you don't have to stop yourself from eating the foods you love, and this can also include various high-fat foods. However, the things that you would normally eat while on a diet may need to be avoided. Here is a list of food items you have to avoid when you are on a keto diet.

Sugary Food

Food or beverages that have high sugar content, such as cakes, ice cream, fruit juices, and sodas, need to be avoided. You also need to stay away from milkshakes and any other dessert that contains sugar.

Fruit

When you are on a keto diet, you have to stay off all fruits except for berries, such as blueberries, blackberries, and strawberries. While it is best to eat more of blueberries as they have high antioxidant properties, you need to limit your portion of berries to small amounts.

Beans and Legumes or Lentils

When you are on a keto diet, you need to stay away from beans, legumes, lentils, and chickpeas.

Grains and Starches

Most grains and starches contain a high amount of carbohydrates, which is why you have to stay away from them when you are on a keto diet.

Root Vegetables

All vegetables that grow underground, such as potatoes, sweet potatoes, carrots, turnips, and parsnips, need to be avoided.

Diet Food

Most diet bars and diet foods contain a lot of grains, which are high in carbohydrates. All these diet foods and energy bars should be avoided when you are on a keto diet.

Sauces and Condiments

Sauces and condiments contain a lot of sugar and healthy fat, which is why you should stay away from them. These include mayonnaise and food dips as well as salad dressings that you usually find at the supermarket.

Alcohol

Alcohol has high carbohydrate content, so you have to stay away from alcohol when you are on a keto diet.

Foods to Include in a Keto Diet

Meat

The best part about going on a keto diet is that you can eat any kind of meat, including steak, ham, sausage, bacon, turkey, or chicken, to your heart's content.

Fish

Fish is a great source of protein and healthy fat, which is why you should include salmon, tuna, and mackerel in your keto diet meals.

Eggs

When you are on a keto diet, try to look for omega-3 eggs, which are great to support your body through the diet plan.

Butter and Cream

While you can include butter and cream in proportion, try not to overindulge in it.

Cheese

The dream of every keto diet follower is to eat healthy; however, there's nothing tasty about healthy food. The best part about your keto diet is that you can add cheese to it. Unprocessed cheeses like cheddar, blue cheese, and mozzarella are keto-approved.

Nuts and Seeds

A great way to keep you feeling full during your diet is to eat as many nuts and seeds as possible. You can even fix up a salad by adding a few nuts and seeds to make it tasty and healthy. A keto diet follower should include almonds, walnuts, pumpkin seeds, flax seeds, and even chia seeds to make a smoothie.

Healthy Oils

When you are on a keto diet, try to cook with as much healthy oil as possible, and this doesn't necessarily mean expensive extra-virgin olive oil. While olive oil is great, you can also use coconut oil or even avocado oil, which works just as well.

Low-Carbohydrate Vegetables

When you are on a keto diet, try to eat as much green leafy vegetables. You should also include tomatoes, onions, bell peppers, and capsicum in your diet.

Condiments

If you are worried about adding taste to the food while you are on a keto diet, you can use a large variety of herbs and spices, as well as salt and pepper, to add flavor to your meals.

In order for the keto diet to start working in your favor, it's important for you to activate autophagy. The best way to do this is to go through the tips mentioned in chapter 3 so that you can activate autophagy before you get on to a keto diet for the best results. When followed effectively, not only do you manage to get in amazing shape with this diet, but it works wonders on your skin and hair. It also reverses the signs of aging, not just externally but internally as well.

Chapter 6: Exercise

There are many benefits of exercising, and one of the greatest benefits is being able to activate autophagy. People usually try many things to increase the autophagy process in their body, but they forget that the simplest way to do so is by exercising regularly. Apart from helping activate autophagy, you will also receive a number of benefits from exercising. Here are a few benefits that are extremely crucial and will help your body function in an efficient manner.

Faster Fat Burning

When the metabolism rate in your body goes low, you start to gain weight because your body is not able to process the fats efficiently. Unhealthy accumulation of fats not only makes you gain weight but also puts a lot of stress on the other organs of your body. One of the best ways to lose weight is by increasing the metabolism rate in the body. This can be done by exercising regularly.

While it has been said a million times that exercising helps in losing weight, a number of people do not realize how it actually helps. Exercising regularly will help activate autophagy, and this, in turn, will help increase the metabolism rate. However, you should know how much exercise is good for your body before you reach the stage of muscle damage and cell damage. While autophagy will help repair the cells in the body, if you're overindulgent while exercising, you may end up damaging muscles as well as a lot of cells, and this may be very difficult for autophagy to repair in a short time frame.

Get Fit

Another benefit of exercising regularly is you will look fit and stay healthy. People usually spend hours in the gym, trying to tone up the body and get that slim look that they were craving for. With the help of exercising, you will be able to get this in no time; however, you need to find the right exercises that will help activate autophagy in your body. Simply lifting weights and running on the treadmill may or may not work for you. You need to understand what will help your body and how you can go ahead and activate autophagy efficiently. When you pick the right exercises for your body, you will be able to get a well-toned body in no time, and this will also help with your weight loss process.

Get a Muscular Look

Regular exercise helps you to burn fat and firm up your body. When you are overweight, the skin on your body expands to accommodate the extra fat. When you start losing weight, the skin begins to sag, and it becomes loose. When you combine an effective weight loss diet plan along with exercise, your body tends to firm up a lot faster, and you don't have saggy or loose skin. This helps you look younger and lesser than your actual weight. Regular exercise doesn't necessarily mean you have to spend long hours at the gym. Regular body movement and walks can help your body get in shape to a great extent and help you have a more toned structure.

Great for Your Organs

Regular movement of the body not only

improves your external physique but also helps your vital organs function more effectively. One of the major benefits of exercise is that it helps in improving the autophagy process. This not only works well for metabolic regulation but also benefits the heart, ensuring that it functions well. When your heart starts pumping blood more regularly, there is a lower risk of blockages around the heart as well as clots in various parts of your body that could be dangerous. Regular exercise also keeps your digestive system healthy and more functional. If you have digestive problems, including constipation, this is something that you can solve by activating autophagy through exercise.

It Makes You Feel Great

Sometimes you might have to push yourself to exercise, but at the end of every session, you will feel great no matter how drained out or tired you are. Apart from the obvious benefits of exercise, it also works wonders on your mind. It helps you relax and lets out all the negative energy that is built up inside of you. When you start channeling your energy toward exercise, you focus on the positive aspects of life, and this reflects in your personality.

It helps eliminate the toxins when you sweat, and your skin starts to glow. Exercise can also help you relax, and this helps you get better sleep at night. If you suffer from insomnia or struggle with sleep because of multiple thoughts running through your mind, a quick walk just before bedtime will make you feel great and will help you fall asleep almost instantly.

A well-rested mind is a fresh mind, and this means you will manage to focus on your tasks a lot better. This gives you more confidence toward your work, and you manage to approach situations with a better mindset.

Chapter 7: Reversing Aging

Autophagy works well not only in enhancing weight loss but also in reversing the early signs of aging. Everyone wants to look good, and the first wrinkle is usually the worst nightmare! While some get it in their fifties, it doesn't wait too long for others, and you might end up with the first early signs of aging when you are as young as thirty.

One of the best things about autophagy is that it helps you to reverse the signs of aging and makes you feel good about the way you look. It also helps you to feel a lot younger from within by repairing damaged cells and enhancing their functionality of the body.

The Most Important Anti-Aging Advice

Aging doesn't go down well with everyone. While some people age gracefully, others look like a complete disaster! This may sound a little harsh, but the truth is, if you do not look after yourself and you don't pay attention to your body, it is going to show on your face eventually, as well as your medical reports. Aging isn't just about how you look but how you feel as well. This is why you need to adopt the right methods of anti-aging. Reverse aging instead of using shortcuts that may benefit you for a few months but eventually may throw you completely off track.

If you want to look young and feel young, it is important for you to take care of your body. You don't have to make massive changes in your life. Just a few healthy changes, and you will be on track to looking great and feeling even better.

Skip the Needles

A lot of people look at the reversal of aging and anti-aging as surgical terms and opt for Botox and other forms of surgery to hide the way they look. This may make you look great for a couple of years, and while you may end up fooling the world, you are not fooling yourself. Simply looking younger than you actually are is not going to do the trick. You have to be younger from within as well. The only way you can do that is by adapting to a healthier lifestyle.

If you start living a life that helps repair cell damage, you won't even need to think about surgical procedures to hide those wrinkles because you will not look that old! The problem with surgical anti-aging procedures is that you begin to fool the world, but inside, there is a lot of damage that you haven't even given a thought to because all you are worried about is your appearance.

There are no shortcuts to getting healthy and looking great. Autophagy may take a while, but once it sets in, the benefits are long-term and without any side effect. This is unlike the procedures that you undergo by going under the knife.

Focus on Your Health First

If you want to start feeling younger and looking better, you have to pay attention to your health. People suffering from health problems tend to look older and feel a lot older than they actually are. If you are in your thirties and walking up a flight of stairs leaves you breathless, then there's a problem that you need to address and rectify as soon as possible.

The problem with most people today is that they don't get enough time to exercise because of the number of hours they spend behind their office desk. Careers today can get very demanding, and this leaves people with little time to focus on their personal life. The reason people have begun to lean toward quick weight loss solutions is that they have very little time in hand. They believe that these solutions are the best bet. The truth is, no matter how erratic your schedule is, you will always find time to contribute toward your health as long as you are focused on it. Even if you spend twelve hours at work, getting up every thirty minutes and taking a three- to four-minute walk will help your body tremendously when accompanied by a healthy diet plan.

The healthier you are, the more active you will be, and you won't get sick as much. Being healthy and fit has nothing to do with your biological age. It's about how much cell damage happens in your body and how you feel at the end of the day. There are some fifty-year-olds that can put a twenty-year-old to shame. The difference between the fifty-year-old and the twenty-year-old lies in the strength of the fifty-year-old and the functionality of the internal organs.

Pay Attention to the Details

In order for you to reverse the signs of aging, you have to be honest with yourself and pay attention to the little details in your life. If you fall sick often and you notice that you can't do as many activities as you used to, then this is probably an early warning that you need to get your life in control. One of the major reasons why people fall sick these days and tend to feel a lot older than they actually are is the kind of food that they eat. We don't realize how much of a difference you can make simply by changing your eating habits and incorporating a little exercise daily. No matter how busy you are, making small changes to lead a healthy life is a small price to pay in comparison to falling sick and falling prey to deadly illnesses in the long run.

Don't Be Too Hard on Yourself

When it comes to reversing the signs of aging, there are always going to be disappointments and probably a little denial with regard to how healthy you actually are. What's important is not to be too hard on yourself at this stage and tell yourself that no matter how bad the situation is, with a few modifications in your life, you can be a lot healthier a few years down the line, and you will be proud of what you achieve.

Motivation is really important, and even if it comes in small portions, it is necessary every day. Make sure you keep telling yourself that things will get better and you are working toward it. You don't have to adapt to a strong keto diet or start intermittent fasting immediately because this is not going to do you any good. It's a slow process that needs time so that your body can adjust and gain benefits out of it. There are no shortcuts to becoming healthy and feeling good, but once you begin, make sure you do not turn back. In order for you to do that, you should always have a systematic plan in place. Make sure that you set realistic goals so that you never disappoint yourself.

You Are What You Eat

If you continue to eat a lot of junk food and high-carbohydrate meals, you won't be able to activate autophagy, and this means that your cells will not be repaired efficiently. A keto diet isn't as difficult as it may seem to be. With the trend gaining more popularity, there are a number of restaurants that cater to ketogenic diet meals, specifically for people who are busy and don't have time to prepare one on their own. We live in a date where technology has gotten the better of us. When it comes to getting healthy, it makes a lot of sense to put this technology to good use and look for restaurants that prepare keto meals around you. The benefit of eating ketogenic meals from a restaurant is that you never get bored and you can keep trying different restaurants till you find one that suits your palate. This saves you a lot of time and helps you not to divert away from your diet even when you have a hectic schedule and no time to prepare your own meal.

Taking Your Time to Make Adjustments

Your body needs time to adjust, and the sooner you understand this, the better it is for your health. If you want to reverse the signs of aging, you have to give your body enough time to cope with the changes you make in your lifestyle. Suddenly eliminating carbohydrates from your diet plan may not work as well as you had expected it to, and you need to keep yourself prepared for it. While some people adjust to a keto diet instantly, others may require a little more time to get used to a different diet plan. You have to understand what your body can handle and how much you should change at a time. If you can't deal with a zero-carb diet every day, try eliminating them one meal at a time till your body has adjusted to the diet. While this takes more time, it ensures you do not fall sick, and it helps activate autophagy a lot better.

Forcing yourself to stick to a diet in order to activate autophagy also doesn't really help. If you feel that you are getting sick and you are not able to adjust to a keto diet, you need to come up with something else in order to activate autophagy. As discussed before, there are a number of ways to activate autophagy. While controlling your diet is important, forcing yourself to follow a strict diet when your body cannot adjust is harmful. You need to look at alternative ways of activating autophagy and reversing the signs of aging.

Feeling Good

Once you introduce autophagy into your life, you will start to feel good, and this is the beginning of the cell repair process inside your body. While you notice the obvious signs where you see amazing changes in your skin and your hair, you will also notice your energy levels are increasing. If you have the tendency of catching a cold or getting cough every time the weather changes, this is something you will notice vanishing once autophagy is in full flow in your body.

Age reversal isn't only about how beautiful you look, but it is also about how healthy you feel from within. It's about eliminating the possible illnesses by healthy cell repair and teaching your body to fight infections more effectively and getting stronger. A few changes in your lifestyle are all you need, and with autophagy activated, you will be beautiful inside and outside, and your youthful glow won't fade.

Chapter 8: Weight Loss

There have been a number of different kinds of weight loss programs you may have come across in recent times. From choosing weight loss supplements to enrolling for exercise regimes that may seem completely out of place to adapting to a diet that you may believe works well in your favor, weight loss is something you can't get out of your mind when you are overweight. However, when it comes to losing weight, you need to keep in mind that it's not a temporary solution that you should rely on. Relying on these will help you get to the desired weight before you decide to go back to your old habits.

Weight loss is all about changing the way you look at life and incorporating certain techniques that will benefit you in the long run and keep you healthy from within as well. A common misconception with weight is that if you are not overweight, you are healthy. The truth, however, is people who aren't that heavy may also suffer from a number of health conditions because of damaged cells in their body, and this is why you need to consider leading a healthy lifestyle rather than obsessing over weight loss or weight management. Having said that, adapting to autophagy has a number of benefits, and weight loss is definitely one of them. The only difference between the weight loss program that autophagy has to offer versus other weight loss programs is that autophagy benefits you from within.

Losing Weight for the Looks

The most obvious reason somebody wants to lose weight is to look good. When you are a few pounds overweight, your confidence level automatically starts to drop, and a feeling of inferiority starts to seep in. While you should always be confident about the way you look, if you are not happy with your appearance, you should do something to change it.

There are tons of people who start getting depressed because of their weight mainly because they can't manage to get in shape no matter what they do. The main reason you might not be able to lose weight is because of low metabolism levels. If your metabolism rate is low, no matter how much you diet or starve yourself, you are not going to get in shape. It is important for you to adapt to autophagy so that you start off the process of weight loss and you boost your metabolism rate in order for your body to start burning fat. This is not going to happen overnight, which is why you have to prepare yourself for long-term results. Do not look for shortcuts.

The problem with most weight loss programs today is that they promote weight loss as a trophy for something that you will do for the next thirty days. Simply popping a pill or following a diet plan only for a month to lose weight is the worst thing you can do to yourself. Not only will this affect your body internally, but it will also reflect on your appearance. While some of these weight loss solutions help you to get in shape, they end up giving you horrible skin, tired eyes, and severe hair loss. This is caused because of the lack of nutrients in your system.

If you want to get healthy and you want to do it the right way, you have to give your body time. Autophagy isn't as popular as other quick weight loss solutions because it's not a quick fix. It is a longtime commitment that you have to make, not only so that you look great but also so that you feel amazing from within and you wave goodbye to illnesses.

Losing Weight to Get Healthy

As mentioned earlier, most weight loss solutions are so that you look great physically, but what you really need is one that makes you healthy from within. One of the most important things you need to understand is that losing weight isn't just about looking great but also getting healthy at the same time. In order for you to do that, you have to choose something that benefits your body internally as well as externally. The reason autophagy is so great is that it helps with repairing your body from within, and you will also be able to see the results externally.

The main difference between a short-term weight loss program and the autophagy way of life lies in the name itself. A short-term weight loss solution will give you short-term results, and you will eventually end up gaining weight and suffer from a number of health problems. Once you activate autophagy, not only will you start losing weight, but you'll get healthy, and this is essential in order for you to keep illnesses away.

Autophagy helps you to reverse the signs of aging because it repairs the cells in your body, and this keeps a number of age-related diseases away, making it a long-term and effective solution that grows on you. While it's not the easiest weight loss process to get used to, it is something that you will learn to adapt and manage to incorporate for the rest of your life so that you lead a healthy life and focus on being healthy rather than just looking great.

Conclusion

If you want to get started on autophagy, it is important for you to research in detail about how you can benefit from it in the best possible way and what techniques are going to work for you. Autophagy is a vast subject, and right from intermittent fasting to keto diet, as well as exercising, it's all about finding the rhythm that suits your body the best.

While some people can start intermittent fasting almost instantly, there are others who may have trouble adjusting to a keto diet because of the lack of carbs in their daily meals. If you want autophagy to work well, you have to activate it by taking the right steps and making sure you have a plan to stick to.

While some people look at it as an instant solution and believe that with a diet plan they will manage to get in shape, it's not going to benefit you in any way. If you want autophagy to work well and work effectively, you need to focus on taking the right steps even if it means investing a lot of time and not seeing results for a few weeks.

Unlike strict diet plans and instant workout regimes that promise you results within a month, autophagy sometimes may take a longer time to kick in, but once it's done, you won't need to worry about a number of health problems, including weight issues. Another great thing about adapting to autophagy is that you give your body enough time to understand what the diet is like, and this becomes a habit without realizing various changes that have occurred.

The best part about autophagy is that it boosts your metabolism, and it works wonders on your digestive system. This is really important for the healthy functionality of your system. It also helps in cell repair so that it reverses the signs of aging.

Not only is autophagy a cost-effective way to stay healthy, but it is also beneficial to you in numerous ways. This is why you should definitely consider adapting to an autophagy way of life.

The best part about autophagy is that it won't interfere with your daily routine, and you don't need to plan a go out of the way in order to make it a successful solution. All you need is the willpower and the courage to take that first step toward getting healthy and ensuring that you do not give up on your plan midway. You will soon be on the path to good health and long life.

Adapting to autophagy is not just a trend that is going to stay in your life for a few months and then disappear for good. It is something that you will have with you for the rest of your life—not just because it makes you look good but because it heals you from within! It's time to burn unnecessary fat, treat your body like a temple, and reverse the signs of aging all at once with one simple yet effective solution—autophagy.